A Fitness Guide for Beginners

Written by Joe Blanc

Thanks to all that inspired me to write this book.

1st edition

A Fitness Guide for Beginners is a book about the details of a 5-7 minute workout routine, diet tips for a healthy body and general tips that I have personally tried that work for weight loss etc...

I don't pretend to be a fitness expert but I thought I would write this book based on my 30 of experience in fitness both in what weight lifting exercises worked for me as well as diet tips.

The book is intended for an audience of beginners or working people who don't have the time to research and try what works. These are for people that will know that I have personally tried and found what works for me as well as you.

Exercises

Exercises for most people are a bit confusing. What I can say is that you have to divide your body into parts. Yours arms, legs, back and chest. All these parts have to be exercised in order to achieve a fit toned body. What we will cover in this section is some basic exercises for each part of the body.

As far as the arms, your major muscles are biceps,

triceps and delts. You can exercise biceps with bicep curls , triceps with overhead extensions and delts with side and front lateral raises.

As for legs, basic exercises are leg curls, leg extensions, calf raises and squats.

For the back you can do seated rows or pull ups. For the chest basic bench press or push ups will do.

Ideally you will pick upper body exercises one day and lower body the next with a minimum of 4 exercises a week. Each exercise I would do 2-3 sets of between 8-10 reps.

With this type of routine it will only take you

between 5-7 minutes to complete per day and every 2 days you will have completed a total body workout.

Diet

As far as diet goes, I would get a calorie counting app such as my fitness pal. This particular app will count the calories of practically any food and will even give you a weight loss goal to follow. It should be said that not all calories are equal. Such as calories from soda or burgers and fries tend to be turned directly into fat whereas food like fish or chicken with rice and vegetables tend to be digested better and even increase your metabolism.

Also try to stay away
from processed foods not in
a natural state as they tend
to turn directly to fat as well.

Cardio

If you want to build up your wind for climbing stairs or whatever, you will have to do some cardio. A lot of people just do bike riding and that's fine. Other people that go to the gym do treadmill or stairclimber exercises and that's fine. If your in martial arts that is also excellent cardio.

What is also popular now is HIIT training. It stands for high intensity interval training. It involves an exercise like jumping jacks for 30 seconds then walk around but don't sit down for 20-30 seconds and then do squats or some other exercise and repeat for 8-10 times. The idea of this type of cardio is to reduce and burn calories.

Tips

I thought I would share with you a few tips that I found on the internet that I have tried and have worked. These tips have to do with hair loss, hair colour and weight loss.

I have always suffered from thin hair and in the past year I went almost bald. I tried hats and shaving my head but then I decided to do some research. I found a vitamin called biotin was helping a lot of people on YouTube so I bought a bottle at 2500 mcg and took it along with a multi vitamin for one year. Below are pictures of the results.

Also, I found that my hair was going grey. I did some more research and found a remedy of a plant based variety. It was to boil the peels of four potatoes and boil them in 2 cups of water for 15 mins. Then strain the water from the peels a let cool off. When cooled off, apply with clean spronge all over hair. I tried this for 3 days and found all my grey hair was gone.

As far as weight loss, I was always fit but recently I had acquired a bit of fat around the belly that I could not get rid of with all the exercise and diet. Then I tried this remedy I found and it all melted away. Put one teaspoon of cinnamon in a boiling cup of water. Let cool off and and then add a teaspoon of honey. I drank this first thing in the morning and before I went to sleep for a month and my belly fat was gone.

I hope you enjoyed the book and will try at least some of the things out to see if they work for you.

The following pictures are from the beginning of taking biotin and the multi vitamin. The second picture is after 6 months and the third is after one year.

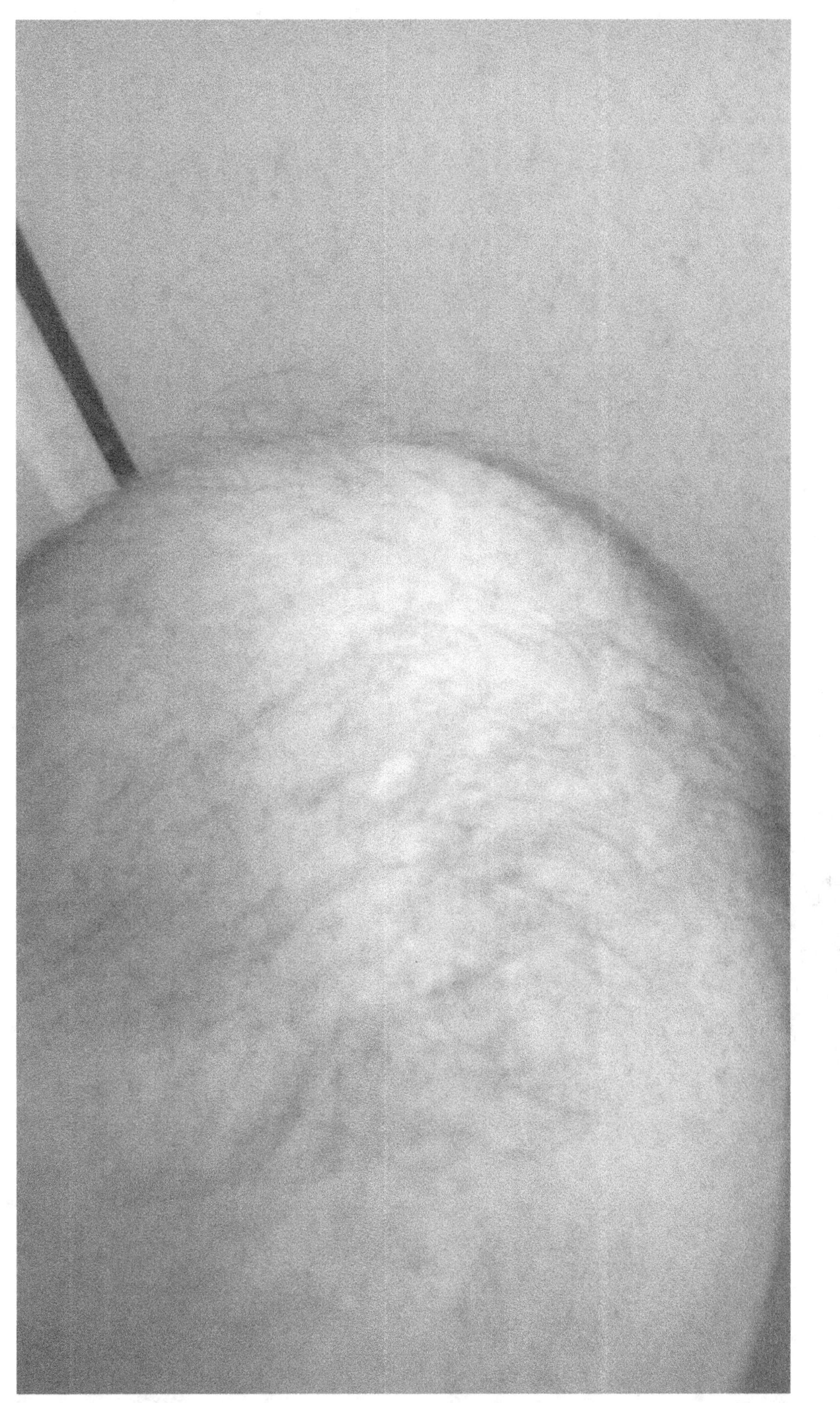

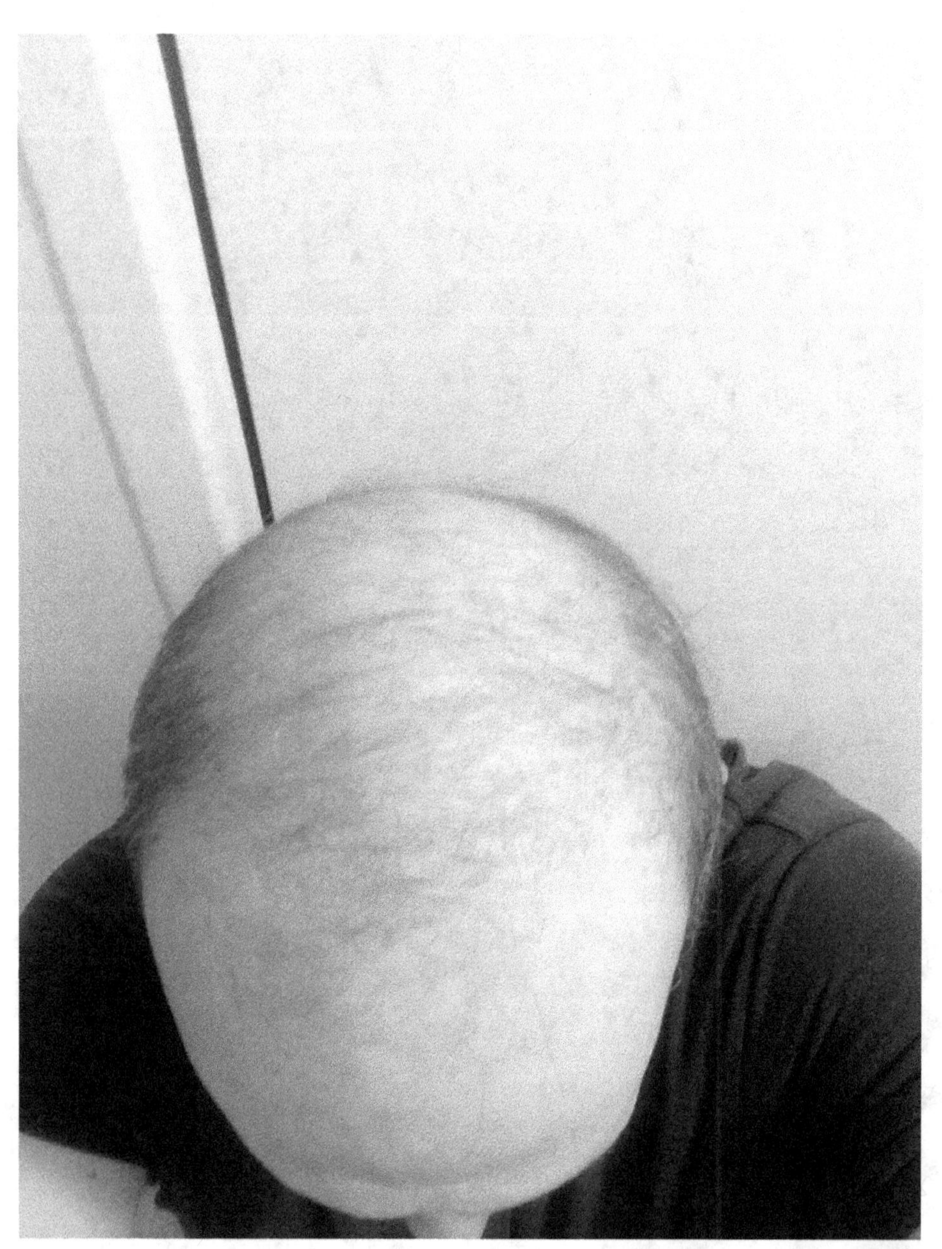

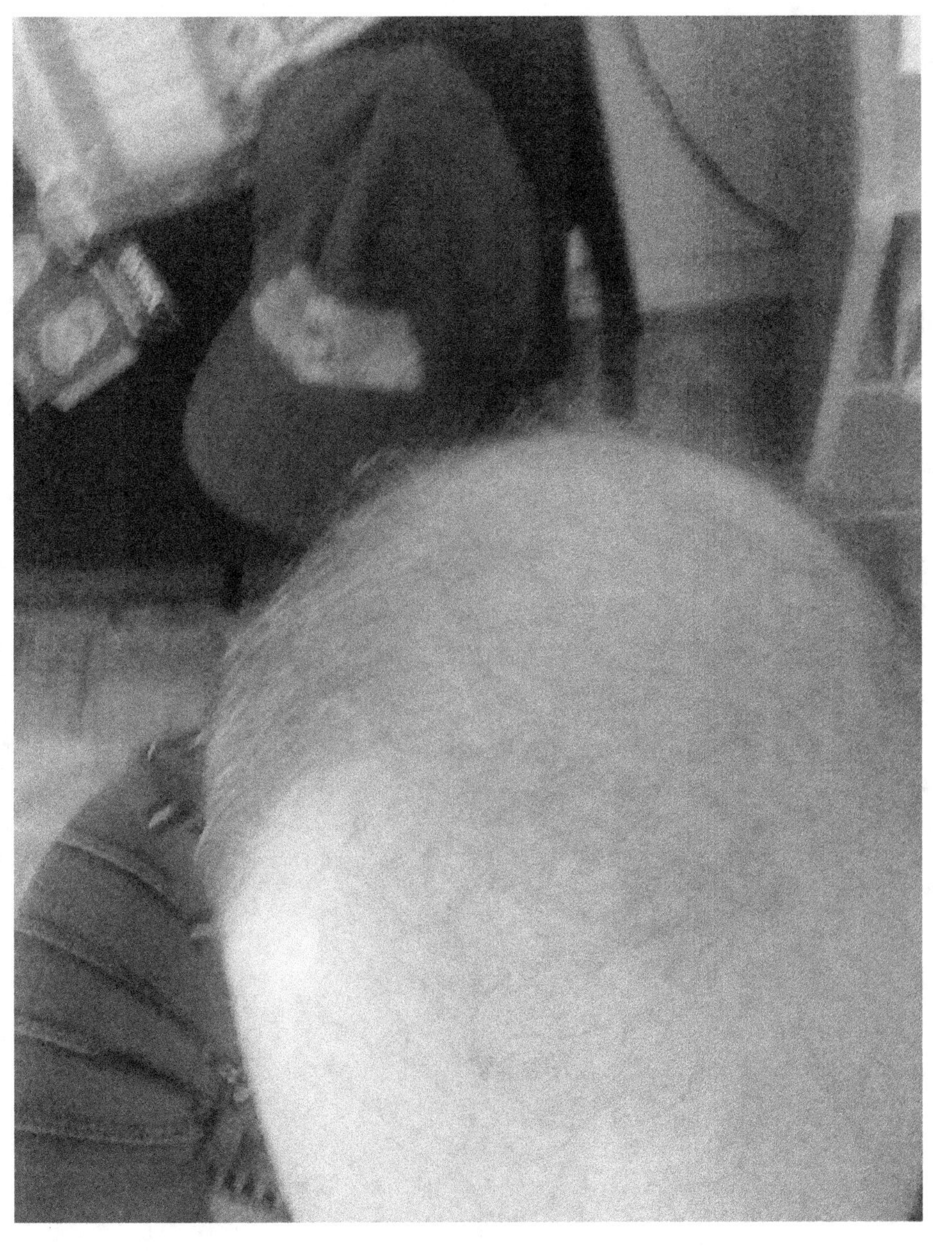

The End